KETO |
COOKBOOK
FOR
BEGINNERS
2021

DISCLAIMER

The information contained in the Book is for informational
urposes only, and in no case may it constitute the formulation of
a diagnosis or the prescription of treatment.
The information contained in the Book is not intended and
should not in any way replace the direct doctor-patient
relationship or the specialist visit.
t is recommended to always seek the advice of your doctor and/
or specialists regarding any indication reported.

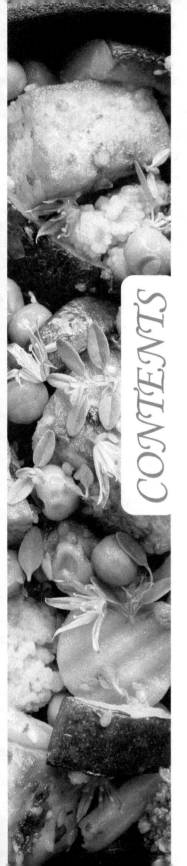

CONTENTS

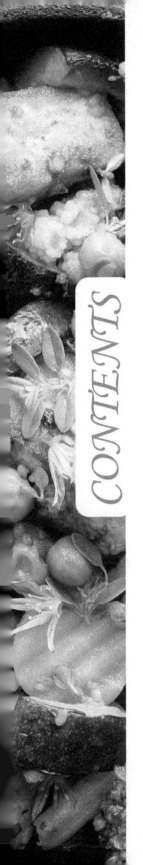

CONTENTS

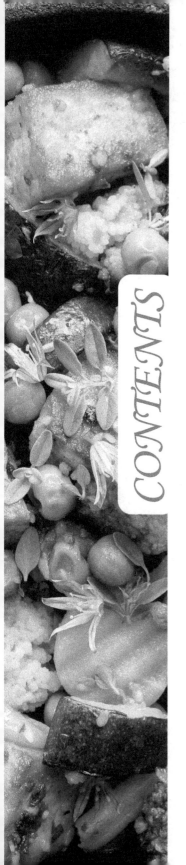

CONTENTS

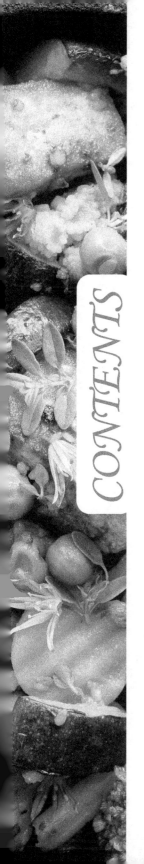

CONTENTS

INTRODUCTION

Is Keto Right for You?

Growing old is part of life, but one can retain an active and healthy lifestyle long into your later years.

The aging process affects the body in many ways. As we age, our bodies undergo a variety of changes. Our hair begins to gray; our skin loses its elasticity, and wrinkles develop. Muscle loss, thinning skin, and reduced stomach acids are all part of the aging process. Most of the changes will make you more susceptible to weight gain while also causing nutrient deficiencies. For example, reduced acids in your stomach can affect how nutrients are being absorbed, such as Iron, Vitamin B2, calcium, and magnesium.

Compounding these issues is that as we age, our bodies require less fuel, and we need to decrease the number of calories we eat in a day. This makes it challenging to make sure we get the nutrients needed while eating fewer calories. It's a bit of a nutritional dilemma.

Lucky for us, there are several steps you can do to prevent deficiencies and other age-related changes. As an example, consuming food that is rich in nutrients and ingesting the right supplements can aid in keeping you healthy as you age. Following a Keto-diet is one great way of staying healthy as you continue to age.

The choices we make regarding our food on a day to day basis and over our lifetime will always matter more than ever. It may occur to you that since the Keto diet does not allow processed foods and carbohydrates that it is a highly restrictive diet. The Keto diet is not restrictive, as far as diet plans go. As long as you stay to the allowed food groups, you will be given free rein to decide what you want to eat. You will not be experiencing boredom since choices of food because there are so many choices available. Here in this book, we will be listing down all the foods you can and can't eat.

Everyone knows that watching what you eat and staying active is vital to a healthy lifestyle. However, as we age, things just aren't that simple. Our nutritional needs evolve. Many women find themselves suffering from physical disorders that can make it difficult to swallow, digest foods properly, or find themselves with a significantly reduced appetite.

Your diet is linked to your immune function; it influences mental health and is critical in maintaining healthy bones and sharp eyes. That means women over 50 should make eating a healthy diet suited to their specific needs the highest priority. Developing and implementing a Keto-friendly diet plan will help to ensure that you are eating nutrient-rich foods while eliminating calorie-dense foods that hold no nutritional value. Because of its focus on eating nutrient-dense foods, the Keto diet is perfect for women over 50. With some tweaking and a few minor adjustments to reduce caloric intake and different nutritional needs, this diet can be tailored to meet everyone's individual needs.

BENEFITS OF KETO DIET

The Keto diet has become so popular in recent years because of the success people have noticed. Not only have they lost weight, but scientific studies show that the Keto diet can help you improve your health in many others. As when starting any new diet or exercise routine, there may seem to be some disadvantages, so we will go over those for the Keto diet. But most people agree that the benefits outweigh the change period!

BENEFITS/ ADVANTAGES

Losing weight: for most people, this is the foremost benefit of switching to Keto! Their previous diet method may have stalled for them, or they were noticing weight creeping back on. With Keto, studies have shown that people have been able to follow this diet and relay fewer hunger pangs and suppressed appetite while losing weight at the same time! You are minimizing your carbohydrate intake, which means more occasional blood sugar spikes.
Often, those fluctuations in blood sugar levels make you feel hungrier and more prone to snacking in between meals.

Instead, by guiding the body towards ketosis, you are eating a more fulfilling diet of fat and protein and harnessing energy from ketone molecules instead of glucose.
Studies show that low-carb diets effectively reduce visceral fat

(the fat you commonly see around the abdomen increases as you become obese).

This reduces your risk of obesity and improves your health in the long run.

REDUCE THE RISK OF TYPE 2 DIABETES:

The problem with carbohydrates is how unstable they make blood sugar levels. This can be very dangerous for people who have diabetes or are pre-diabetic because of unbalanced blood sugar levels or family history.

Keto is an excellent option because of the minimal intake of carbohydrates it requires. Instead, you are harnessing most of your calories from fat or protein, which will not cause blood sugar spikes and, ultimately, less pressured the pancreas to secrete insulin. Many studies have found that diabetes patients who followed the Keto diet lost more weight and eventually reduced their fasting glucose levels. This is monumental news for patients with unstable blood sugar levels or hopes to avoid or reduce their diabetes medication intake.

IMPROVE CARDIOVASCULAR RISK SYMPTOMS TO LOWER YOUR CHANCES OF HAVING HEART DISEASE:

Most people assume that following Keto is so high in fat content has to increase your risk of coronary heart disease or heart attack. But the research proves otherwise! Research shows that switching to Keto can lower your blood pressure, increase your HDL good cholesterol, and reduce your triglyceride fatty acid levels. That's because the fat you are consuming on Keto s healthy and high-quality fats, so they reverse many unhealthy symptoms of heart disease.

hey boost your "good" HDL cholesterol numbers and decrease our "bad" LDL cholesterol numbers. It also reduces the level f triglyceride fatty acids in the bloodstream. A top-level of hese can lead to stroke, heart attack, or premature death. nd what are the top levels of fatty acids linked to?

IGH CONSUMPTION OF CARBOHYDRATES:

Vith the Keto diet, you are drastically cutting your intake of arbohydrates to improve fatty acid levels and improve other sk factors. A 2018 study on the Keto diet found that it can nprove 22 out of 26 risk factors for cardiovascular heart isease! These factors can be critical to some people, especially iose who have a history of heart disease in their family.

ICREASES THE BODY'S ENERGY LEVELS:

et's briefly compare the difference between the glucose iolecules synthesized from a high carbohydrate intake versus etones produced on the Keto diet. The liver makes ketones id use fat molecules you already stored. This makes them uch more energy-rich and an endless source of fuel compared glucose, a simple sugar molecule. These ketones can give iu a burst of energy physically and mentally, allowing you to ive greater focus, clarity, and attention to detail.

DECREASES INFLAMMATION IN THE BODY:

Inflammation on its own is a natural response by the body's immune system, but when it becomes uncontrollable, it can lead to an array of health problems, some severe and some minor The health concerns include acne, autoimmune conditions arthritis, psoriasis, irritable bowel syndrome, and even acne and eczema. Often, removing sugars and carbohydrates from your diet can help patients of these diseases avoid flare-ups and the delightful news is Keto does just that!

A 2008 research study found that Keto decreased a blood marker linked to high inflammation in the body by nearly 40%. This is glorious news for people who may suffer from inflammatory disease and want to change their diet to improve

INCREASES YOUR MENTAL FUNCTIONING LEVEL:

As we elaborated earlier, the energy-rich ketones can boost the body's physical and mental levels of alertness. Research has shown that Keto is a much better energy source for the brain than simple sugar glucose molecules are. With nearly 75% of your diet coming from healthy fats, the brain's neural cell and mitochondria have a better source of energy to function at the highest level.

Some studies have tested patients on the Keto diet and found they had higher cognitive functioning, better memory recall and were less susceptible to memory loss. The Keto diet ca

ven decrease the occurrence of migraines, which can be very
etrimental to patients.

ECREASES RISK OF DISEASES LIKE ALZHEIMER'S, ARKINSON'S, AND EPILEPSY.

hey created the Keto diet in the 1920s to combat epilepsy
children. From there, research has found that Keto can
nprove your cognitive functioning level and protect brain
lls from injury or damage.

lis is very good to reduce the risk of neurodegenerative
sease, which begins in the brain because of neural cells
utating and functioning with damaged parts or lower
an peak optimal functioning. Studies have found that the
llowing Keto can improve the mental functioning of patients
10 suffer from diseases like Alzheimer's or Parkinson's. These
:urodegenerative diseases sadly have no cure, but the Keto
et could improve symptoms as they progress. Researchers
lieve that it's because of cutting out carbs from your diet,
1ich reduces the occurrence of blood sugar spikes that the
·dy's neural cells have to keep adjusting to.

TO CAN REGULATE HORMONES IN WOMEN WHO VE PCOS (POLYCYSTIC OVARY SYNDROME) AND PMS RE-MENSTRUAL SYNDROME).

omen who have PCOS suffer from infertility, which can be
·y heartbreaking for young couples trying to start a family.
r this condition, there is no known cure, but we believe it's
ated to many similar diabetic symptoms like obesity and a

high level of insulin. This causes the body to produce more se[x]
hormones, which can lead to infertility. The Keto diet paved it[s]
way as a popular way to regulate insulin and hormone level[s]
and increase a woman's chances of getting pregnant.

DISADVANTAGES

YOUR BODY WILL HAVE A CHANGED PERIOD:

It depends from person to person on the number of days th[at]
will be, but when you start any new diet or exercise routin[e]
your body has to adjust to the new normal. With the Keto die[t]
you are drastically cutting your carbohydrates intake, so th[e]
body must adjust to that. You may feel slow, weak, exhauste[d]
and like you are not thinking as quick or fast as you used to. [This]
just means that your body is making adjustments to Keto, an[d]
once this change period is done, you will see the weight lo[ss]
results you expected.

IF YOU ARE AN ATHLETE, YOU MAY NEED MOR[E] CARBOHYDRATES:

If you still want to try Keto as an athlete, you must talk [to]
your nutritionist or trainer to see how the diet can be tweak[ed]
for you. Most athletes require a greater intake of carbs th[an]
the Keto diet requires, which means they may have to [up]
their intake to ensure they have the energy for their traini[ng]
sessions.

High endurance sports (like rugby or soccer) and hea[vy]
weightlifting require more significant information [on]
carbohydrates. If you're an athlete wanting to follow Ke[to]

nd gain the health benefits, it's crucial you first talk to your rainer before changing your diet.

OU HAVE TO COUNT YOUR DAILY MACROS CAREFULLY:

or beginners, this can be tough, and even people already n Keto can become lazy about this. People are often used to ating what they want without worrying about just how many rams of protein or carbs it contains.

/ith Keto, be meticulous about counting your intake to nsure you are maintaining the Keto breakdown (75% fat, 20% rotein, ~5% carbs). The closer you stick to this, the better esults you will see regarding weight loss and other health enefits. If your weight loss has stalled or you're not feeling s energetic as you hoped, it could be because your macros e off. Find a free calorie counting app that you look at the gredients of everything you're eating and cooking.

_____

BREAKFAST RECIPES

Cheesy Breakfast Muffins

Preparation Time: 15 minutes

Cooking Time: 12 minutes

Servings: 6

Ingredients:

4 tablespoons melted butter

3/4 tablespoon baking powder

1 cup almond flour

2 large eggs, lightly beaten

2 ounces cream cheese mixed with 2 tablespoons heavy whipping cream

A handful of shredded Mexican blend cheese

Directions:

Preheat the oven to 400°F. Grease 6 muffin tin cups with melted butter and set aside.

Combine the baking powder and almond flour in a bowl. Stir well and set aside.

Stir together four tablespoons melted butter, eggs, shredded cheese, and cream cheese in a separate bowl.

The egg and the dry mixture must be combined using a hand mixer to beat until it is creamy and well blended.

The mixture must be scooped into the greased muffin cups evenly.

Baking time: 12 minutes

Nutrition:

Calories: 214

Fat: 15.6g

Fiber: 3.1g

Carbohydrates: 5.1 g

Protein: 9.5 g

Spinach, Mushroom, and Goat Cheese Frittata

Preparation Time: 15 minutes

Cooking Time: 20 minutes

Servings: 5

Ingredients:

2 tablespoons olive oil

1 cup fresh mushrooms, sliced

6 bacon slices, cooked and chopped

1 cup spinach, shredded

10 large eggs, beaten

1/2 cup goat cheese, crumbled

Pepper and salt

Directions:

Preheat the oven to 350°F.

Heat oil and add the mushrooms and fry for 3 minutes until they start to brown, stirring frequently.

Add in the bacon and spinach and cook for about 1 to 2 minutes, or until spinach is wilted.

Slowly pour in the beaten eggs and cook for 3 to 4 minutes. Making use of a spatula, lift the edges for allowing uncooked egg to flow underneath.

Top with the goat cheese, then sprinkle the salt and pepper to season.

Bake in the preheated oven for about 15 minutes until lightly golde
brown around the edges.

Nutrition:

Calories: 265

Fat: 11.6g

Fiber: 8.6g

Carbohydrates: 5.1 g

Protein: 12.9g

Yogurt Waffles

Ingredients:

1/2 cup golden flax seeds meal

1/2 cup plus 3 tablespoons almond flour

1-11/2 tablespoons granulated Erythritol

1 tablespoon unsweetened vanilla whey protein powder

1/4 teaspoon baking soda

1/2 teaspoon organic baking powder

1/4 teaspoon xanthan gum

Salt, as required

1 large organic egg, white and yolk separated

1 organic whole egg

2 tablespoons unsweetened almond milk

11/2 tablespoons unsalted butter

3 ounces plain Greek yogurt

Directions:

Preheat the waffle iron and then grease it.

In a large bowl, add the flour, Erythritol, protein powder, baking soda, baking powder, xanthan gum, salt, and mix until well combined.

In another bowl or container, put in the egg white and beat until stiff peaks form.

In a third bowl, add two egg yolks, whole egg, almond milk, butter, yogurt, and beat until well combined.

Place egg mixture into the bowl of the flour mixture and mix until well combined.

Gently, fold in the beaten egg whites.

Place 1/4 cup of the mixture into preheated waffle iron and cook for about 4–5 minutes or until golden brown.

Repeat with the remaining mixture.

Serve warm.

Nutrition:

Calories: 265

Fat: 11.5g

Fiber: 9.5g

Carbohydrates: 5.2g

Protein: 7.5g

Green Vegetable Quiche

Preparation Time: 20 minutes

Cooking Time: 20 minutes

Servings: 4

Ingredients:

6 organic eggs

1/2 cup unsweetened almond milk

Salt and ground black pepper, as required

2 cups fresh baby spinach, chopped

1/2 cup green bell pepper, seeded and chopped

1 scallion, chopped

1/4 cup fresh cilantro, chopped

1 tablespoon fresh chives, minced

3 tablespoons mozzarella cheese, grated

Directions:

Preheat your oven to 400°F.

Lightly grease a pie dish.

In a bowl, add eggs, almond milk, salt, and black pepper, and beat until well combined. Set aside.

In another bowl, add the vegetables and herbs and mix well.

At the bottom of the prepared pie dish, place the veggie mixture evenly and top with the egg mixture.

Let the quiche bake for about 20 minutes.

Remove the pie dish from the oven and immediately sprinkle with the Parmesan cheese.

Set aside for about 5 minutes before slicing.

Cut into desired sized wedges and serve warm.

Nutrition:

Calories: 298

Fat: 10.4g

Fiber: 5.9g

Carbohydrates: 4.1 g

Protein: 7.9g

Cheesy Broccoli Muffins

Preparation Time: 15 minutes

Cooking Time: 20 minutes

Servings: 6

Ingredients:

2 tablespoons unsalted butter

6 large organic eggs

1/2 cup heavy whipping cream

1/2 cup Parmesan cheese, grated

Salt and ground black pepper, as required

11/4 cups broccoli, chopped

2 tablespoons fresh parsley, chopped

1/2 cup Swiss cheese, grated

Directions:

Grease a 12-cup muffin tin.

In a bowl or container, put in the cream, eggs, Parmesan cheese, salt, and black pepper, and beat until well combined.

Divide the broccoli and parsley in the bottom of each prepared muffin cup evenly.

Top with the egg mixture, followed by the Swiss cheese.

Let the muffins bake for about 20 minutes, rotating the pan once halfway through.

Carefully, invert the muffins onto a serving platter and serve warm.

Nutrition:

Calories: 241

Fat: 11.5g

Fiber: 8.5g

Carbohydrates: 4.1 g

Protein: 11.1g

Berry Chocolate Breakfast Bowl

Preparation Time: 10 minutes

Cooking Time: 0 minutes

Servings: 2

Ingredients:

1/2 cup strawberries, fresh or frozen

1/2 cup blueberries, fresh or frozen

1 cup unsweetened almond milk

Sugar-free maple syrup to taste

2 tbsp. unsweetened cocoa powder

1 tbsp. cashew nuts for topping

Directions:

The berries must be divided into four bowls, pour on the almond milk.

Drizzle with the maple syrup and sprinkle the cocoa powder on top, a tablespoon per bowl.

Top with the cashew nuts and enjoy immediately.

Nutrition:

Calories: 287

Fat: 5.9g

Fiber: 11.4g

Carbohydrates: 3.1 g

Protein: 4.2g

Goat Cheese Frittata

Preparation Time: 15 minutes

Cooking Time: 15 minutes

Servings: 4

Ingredients:

- 1 tbsp. avocado oil for frying
- 2 oz. (56 g) bacon slices, chopped
- 1 red bell pepper
- 1 small yellow onion, chopped
- 2 scallions, chopped
- 1 tbsp. chopped fresh chives
- Salt and black pepper to taste
- 8 eggs, beaten
- 1 tbsp. unsweetened almond milk
- 1 tbsp. chopped fresh parsley
- 3 1/2 oz. (100 g) goat cheese, divided
- 3/4 oz. (20 g) grated Parmesan cheese

Directions:

Let the oven preheat to 350°F/175°C.

Heat the avocado oil in a medium cast-iron pan and cook the bacon minutes or golden brown. Stir in the bell pepper, onion, scallions, and hives.

Cook for 3 to 4 minutes or until the vegetables soften. Season with salt and black pepper.

In a bowl or container, the eggs must be beaten with the almond milk and parsley.

Pour the mixture over the vegetables, stirring to spread out nicely. Share half of the goat cheese on top.

Once the eggs start to set, divide the remaining goat cheese on top, season with salt, black pepper, and place the pan in the oven—Bake for 5 to 6 minutes or until the eggs set all around.

Take out the pan, scatter the Parmesan cheese on top, slice, and serve warm.

Nutrition:

Calories: 412

Fat: 15.4g

Fiber: 11.2g

Carbohydrates: 4.9 g

Protein: 10.5g

Fluffy Chocolate Pancakes

Preparation Time: 15 minutes

Cooking Time: 12 minutes

Servings: 4

Ingredients:

- 2 cups (250 g) almond flour

- 2 tsp. baking powder

- 2 tbsp... Erythritol

- 3/4 tsp. salt

- 2 eggs

- 1 1/3 cups (320 ml) almond milk

- 2 tbsp. butter + more for frying

Topping:

- 2 tbsp. unsweetened chocolate buttons

- Sugar-free maple syrup

- 4 tbsp. semi-salted butter

Directions:

In a bowl or container, mix the almond flour, baking powder, Erythritol and salt.

Whisk the eggs, almond milk, and butter in another bowl.

ombine in the dry ingredients and mix well.

Ielt about 1 1/2 tablespoon of butter in a non-stick skillet, pour in ortions of the batter to make small circles, about two pieces per batch pproximately 1/4 cup of batter each).

orinkle some chocolate buttons on top and cook for 1 to 2 minutes or otil set beneath.

orn the pancakes and cook for one more minute or until set.

emove the pancakes onto a plate and make more with the remaining gredients.

ork with more butter and reduce the heat as needed to prevent sticking d burning.

izzle the pancakes with some maple syrup, top with more butter (as sired), and enjoy!

utrition:

lories: 384

t: 12.9g

oer: 5.4g

rbohydrates: 7.5 g

Almond Banana Bread

Preparation time: 10 minutes

Cooking time: 4 hours

Servings: 2

Ingredients:

- 1 egg

- 2 tablespoons butter, melted

- ½ cup sugar

- 1 cup flour

- ½ teaspoon baking powder

- ¼ teaspoon baking soda

- A pinch of cinnamon powder

- A pinch of nutmeg, ground

- 2 bananas, mashed

- ¼ cup almonds, sliced

- Cooking spray

Directions:

In a bowl, mix sugar with flour, baking powder, baking soda, cinnam
and nutmeg and stir.

Add egg, butter, almonds and bananas and stir really well.

Grease your slow cooker with cooking spray, pour bread mix, cover and cook on Low for 4 hours.

Slice bread and serve for breakfast.

Enjoy!

Nutrition

Calories 211,

Fat 3,

Fiber 6,

Carbs 12,

Protein 5

Sage Potato Casserole

Preparation time: 10 minutes

Cooking time: 3 hours and 30 minutes

Servings: 2

Ingredients:

- 1 teaspoon onion powder
- 2 eggs, whisked
- ½ teaspoon garlic powder
- ½ teaspoon sage, dried
- Salt and black pepper to the taste
- ½ yellow onion, chopped
- 1 tablespoons parsley, chopped
- 2 garlic cloves, minced
- A pinch of red pepper flakes
- ½ tablespoon olive oil
- 2 red potatoes, cubed

Directions:

Grease your slow cooker with the oil, add potatoes, onion, garlic, parsl and pepper flakes and toss a bit.

In a bowl, mix eggs with onion powder, garlic powder, sage, salt a pepper, whisk well and pour over potatoes.

Cover, cook on High for 3 hours and 30 minutes, divide into 2 plates and serve for breakfast.

Enjoy!

Nutrition:

Calories 218,

Fat 6,

Fiber 6,

Carbs 14, Protein 5

Cheddar Hash Browns

Preparation time: 10 minutes

Cooking time: 3 hours

Servings: 2

Ingredients:

- 1 tablespoon butter
- 2 tablespoons mushrooms, chopped
- 2 tablespoons yellow onion, chopped
- ¼ teaspoon garlic powder
- 1 tablespoon flour
- ½ cup milk
- ¼ cup sour cream
- 10 ounces hash browns
- ¼ cup cheddar cheese, shredded
- Salt and black pepper to the taste
- ½ tablespoon parsley, chopped
- Cooking spray

Directions:

Heat up a pan with the butter over medium heat, add onion and mushroom garlic powder and flour, stir and cook for 1 minute.

dd milk gradually, stir, cook until it thickens and take off heat.

rease your slow cooker with cooking spray and add mushrooms mix.

dd hash browns, sour cream, cheddar cheese, salt and pepper, cover and ook on High for 3 hours. Divide between plates and serve right away for eakfast with parsley sprinkled on top Enjoy!

utrition:

ilories 245,

it 4,

ber 7,

irbs 7,

otein 10

Cream Cheese Banana Breakfast

Preparation time: 10 minutes

Cooking time: 4 hours

Servings: 2

Ingredients:

- ½ French baguette, sliced

- 2 bananas, sliced

- 2 ounces cream cheese

- 1 tablespoon brown sugar

- ¼ cup walnuts, chopped

- 1 egg, whisked

- 3 tablespoons skim milk

- 2 tablespoons honey

- ½ teaspoon cinnamon powder

- A pinch of nutmeg, ground

- ¼ teaspoon vanilla extract

- 1 tablespoon butter Cooking spray

Directions:

Spread cream cheese on all bread slices and grease your slow cooker w
cooking spray.

Arrange bread slices in your slow cooker, layer banana slices, brown sugar and walnuts.

In a bowl, mix eggs with skim milk, honey, cinnamon, nutmeg and vanilla extract, and whisk and add over bread slices.

Add butter, cover, cook on Low for 4 hours, divide between plates and serve for breakfast.

Enjoy!

Nutrition:

Calories 251,

Fat 5,

Fiber 7,

Carbs 12, Protein 4

Peanut Butter Oatmeal

Preparation time: 10 minutes

Cooking time: 8 hours

Servings: 2

Ingredients:

- 1 banana, mashed

- 1 and ½ cups almond milk

- ½ cup steel cut oats

- 2 tablespoons peanut butter

- ½ teaspoon vanilla extract

- ½ teaspoon cinnamon powder ½ tablespoon chia seeds

Directions:

In your slow cooker, mix almond milk with banana, oats, peanut butte
vanilla extract, cinnamon and chia, stir, cover and cook on Low for
hours.

Stir oatmeal one more time, divide into 2 bowls and serve.

Enjoy!

Nutrition:

Calories 222,

Fat 5,

Fiber 6,

Carbs 9,

Protein 11

Chocolate Toast

Preparation time: 15 minutes

Cooking time: 40 minutes

Servings: 4

Ingredients:

4 white bread slices

1 tablespoon vanilla extract

2 tablespoons Novella

1 banana, mashed

1 tablespoon coconut oil

¼ cup full-fat milk

Direction

Mix vanilla extract, Novella, mashed banana, coconut oil, and milk.

Pour the mixture in the slow cooker and cook on High for 40 minutes.

Make a quick pressure release and cool the chocolate mixture.

Spread the toasts with cooked mixture.

Nutrition:
8 calories,
 protein,
.2g carbohydrates,
 g fat,
 g fiber,
 g cholesterol,
 mg sodium,
 2mg potassium.

Sweet potato breakfast pie

Preparation time: 10 minutes

Cooking time: 7 hours

Servings: 6

Ingredients:

- 1 shredded sweet potato (peeled)

- 1 pound turkey bacon

- 9 eggs

- 1 small diced sweet onion

- 1 tsp. cinnamon

- 1 tsp. dried basil

- Salt and pepper

Directions:

Grease your slow cooker as you would a baking dish.

Shred the sweet potato and get all ingredients ready.

Cut the bacon into small pieces.

Then whisk the eggs and add all the ingredients into the slow cooker.

Cook on low temperature for 7 to 8 hours.

You can serve it as a pie, by cutting slices or like a cake cutting squares

Nutrition:

245 Cal,

11.5 g total fat (4.6 g sat. fat), 152 mg chop. 189 mg sodium,

7.5 g carb. , 3.9g fiber, , 9.6. G protein.

Fried Apple Slices

Preparation time: 10 minutes

Cooking time: 6 hours

Servings: 6

Ingredients:

1 teaspoon ground cinnamon

3 tablespoons cornstarch

3 pounds Granny Smith apples

¼ teaspoon nutmeg, freshly grated

1 cup sugar, granulated

2 tablespoons butter

Directions:

Put the apple slices in the crock pot and stir in nutmeg, cinnamon, sugar and cornstarch.

Top with butter and cover the lid.

Cook on LOW for about 6 hours, stirring about halfway.

Dish out to serve hot.

Nutrition

Calories: 234

Fat: 4.1g ,Carbohydrates: 52.7g

Banana & Blueberry Oats

Preparation time: 10 minutes

Cooking time: 6 hours

Servings: 2

Ingredients:

- 1/2 cup steel cut oats

- ¼ cup quinoa

- ½ cup blueberries 1 banana, mashed

- A pinch of cinnamon powder

- 2 tablespoons maple syrup

- 2 cups water

- Cooking spray ½ cup coconut milk

Directions:

Grease your slow cooker with cooking spray, add oats, quinoa, blueberri
banana, cinnamon, maple syrup, water and coconut milk, stir, cover a
cook on Low for 6 hours.

Divide into 2 bowls and serve for breakfast.

Enjoy!

Nutrition:

Calories 200, Fat 4, Fiber 5, Carbs 8, Protein 5

Pear and Maple Oatmeal

Preparation time: 10 minutes

Cooking time: 7 hours

Servings: 2

Ingredients:

1 and ½ cups milk

½ cup steel cut oats

½ teaspoon vanilla extract

1 pear, chopped

½ teaspoon maple extract

1 tablespoon sugar

Directions:

In your slow cooker, combine milk with oats, vanilla, pear, maple extract and sugar, stir, cover and cook on Low for 7 hours.

Divide into bowls and serve for breakfast.

Enjoy!

Nutrition:

Calories 200,

Fat 5,

Fiber 7,

Carbs 14, Protein 4

Almond & Strawberry Oatmeal

Preparation time: 10 minutes

Cooking time: 6 hours

Servings: 2

Ingredients:

- 1 cup steel cut oats

- 3 cups water

- 1 cup almond milk

- 1 cup strawberries, chopped

- ½ cup Greek yogurt

- ½ teaspoon cinnamon powder ½ teaspoon vanilla extract

Directions:

In your slow cooker, mix oats with water, milk, strawberries, yogu cinnamon and vanilla, toss, cover and cook on Low for 6 hours.

Stir your oatmeal one more time, divide into bowls and serve for breakfa

Enjoy!

Nutrition:

Calories 201,

Fat 3,

Fiber 6, Carbs 12, Protein 6

Coconut Raisins Oatmeal

Preparation time: 10 minutes

Cooking time: 8 hours

Servings: 2

Ingredients:

½ cup water

½ cup coconut milk

½ cup steel cut oats

½ cup carrots, grated

¼ cup raisins

A pinch of cinnamon powder

A pinch of ginger, ground

A pinch of nutmeg, ground

¼ cup coconut flakes, shredded

1 tablespoon orange zest, grated

½ teaspoon vanilla extract ½ tablespoon maple syrup 2 tablespoons walnuts, chopped

Directions:

your slow cooker, mix water with coconut milk, oats, carrots, raisins, cinnamon, ginger, nutmeg, coconut flakes, orange zest, vanilla extract and maple syrup, stir, cover and cook on Low for 8 hours.

Add walnuts, stir, divide into 2 bowls and serve for breakfast.

Enjoy!

Nutrition:

Calories 200,

Fat 4,

Fiber 6,

Carbs 8,

Protein 8

Cauliflower with Eggs

Preparation time: 10 minutes

Cooking time: 7 hours

Servings: 2

Ingredients:

Cooking spray

4 eggs, whisked

A pinch of salt and black pepper

¼ teaspoon thyme, dried

½ teaspoon turmeric powder

1 cup cauliflower florets

½ small yellow onion, chopped

3 ounces breakfast sausages, sliced

½ cup cheddar cheese, shredded

Directions:

Grease your slow cooker with cooking spray and spread the cauliflower florets on the bottom of the pot.

Add the eggs mixed with salt, pepper and the other ingredients and toss.

Put the lid on, cook on Low for 7 hours, divide between plates and serve for breakfast.

Nutrition:

Calories 261, Fat 6, Fiber 7, Carbs 22, Protein 6

Caramel Pecan Sticky Buns

Preparation time: 40 minutes

Cooking time: 2 hours

Servings: 4

Ingredients:

- ¾ cup packed brown sugar

- 15 ounces refrigerated biscuits

- 1 teaspoon ground cinnamon

- 6 tablespoons melted butter ¼ cup pecans, finely chopped

Directions:

Mix together brown sugar, cinnamon and chopped nuts in a bowl.

Dip refrigerator biscuits in melted butter to coat, then in the brown sug mixture.

Grease a crockpot and layer the biscuits in the crock pot.

Top with the remaining brown sugar mixture and cover the lid.

Cook on HIGH for about 2 hours and dish out to serve.

Nutrition

Calories: 583

Fat: 23.5g

Carbohydrates: 86.2g

Vegetable Omelet

Preparation time: 10 minutes

Cooking time: 2 hours

Servings: 2

Ingredients

6 eggs

½ cup milk

¼ teaspoon salt

Black pepper, to taste

1/8 teaspoon garlic powder

1/8 teaspoon chili powder

1 cup broccoli florets

1 red bell pepper, thinly sliced

1 small yellow onion, finely chopped

1 garlic clove, minced

For Garnishing

Chopped tomatoes

Fresh parsley

Shredded cheddar cheese

Chopped onions

Directions:

Mix together eggs, milk, garlic powder, chili powder, salt and black pepper in a large mixing bowl.

Grease a crockpot and add garlic, onions, broccoli florets and sliced peppers.

Stir in the egg mixture and cover the lid.

Cook on HIGH for about 2 hours.

Top with cheese and allow it to stand for about 3 minutes.

Dish out the omelet into a serving plate and garnish with chopped onion chopped tomatoes and fresh parsley.

Nutrition

Calories: 136

Fat: 7.4g

Carbohydrates: 7.8g

Chia Oatmeal

Preparation time: 10 minutes

Cooking time: 8 hours

Servings: 2

Ingredients:

  2 cups almond milk

  1 cup steel cut oats

  2 tablespoons butter, soft

  ½ teaspoon almond extract

  2 tablespoons chia seeds

Directions:

  your slow cooker, mix the oats with the chia seeds and the other
gredients, toss, put the lid on and cook on Low for 8 hours.

ir the oatmeal one more time, divide into 2 bowls and serve.

Nutrition:

Calories 812,

t 71.4,

ber 9.4,

rbs 41.1,

otein 11

Vanilla Pumpkin Bread

Preparation time: 10 minutes

Cooking time: 2 hours

Servings: 2

Ingredients:

- Cooking spray
- ½ cup white flour
- ½ cup whole wheat flour
- ½ teaspoon baking soda
- A pinch of cinnamon powder
- 2 tablespoons olive oil
- 2 tablespoons maple syrup
- 1 egg
- ½ tablespoon milk
- ½ teaspoon vanilla extract
- ½ cup pumpkin puree
- 2 tablespoons walnuts, chopped
- 2 tablespoons chocolate chips

Directions:

In a bowl, mix white flour with whole wheat flour, baking soda a nnamon and stir.

dd maple syrup, olive oil, egg, milk, vanilla extract, pumpkin puree, alnuts and chocolate chips and stir well.

rease a loaf pan that fits your slow cooker with cooking spray, pour umpkin bread, transfer to your cooker and cook on High for 2 hours.

ice bread, divide between plates and serve.

ijoy!

utrition

lories 200,

: 3,

er 5,

rbs 8,

otein 4

Cheddar Sausage Potatoes

Preparation time: 10 minutes

Cooking time: 4 hours

Servings: 2

Ingredients:

- 1 potato, chopped

- ½ red bell pepper, chopped

- ½ green bell pepper, chopped

- ½ yellow onion, chopped

- 4 ounces smoked Andouille sausage, sliced

- 1 cup cheddar cheese, shredded

- ¼ cup sour cream

- A pinch of oregano, dried

- ¼ teaspoon basil, dried

- 4 ounces chicken cream

- Salt and black pepper to the taste

- 1 tablespoon parsley, chopped

Directions:

Put the potato in your slow cooker, add red bell pepper, green bell pepp
onion, sausage, cheese, sour cream, oregano, basil, salt, pepper a

hicken cream, cover and cook on Low for 4 hours.

dd parsley, toss, divide between plates and serve for breakfast.

njoy!

Tutrition:

alories 355,

at 14,

ber 4,

arbs 20,

otein 22

Frittatas for Breakfast

Preparation time: 5 minutes

Cooking time: 2 hours

Servings: 6

Ingredients:

- Black pepper-1/2 tbsp.

- Sausages-1

- Eggs-8 Spinach-3/4 cup Sea salt-1 tsp.

- Bell pepper-1 ½ cups

- Onions-1/4 cup

Directions:

Mix together all the ingredients.

Put them in the slow cooker and let it cook for 2-3 hours.

Serve hot.

Nutrition:

Calories: 590, Total fat: 47g,

Cholesterol: 45 mg, Sodium: 610 mg,

Carbohydrate: 16g, Dietary fiber: 1g,

Protein: 12g

Easy Buttery Oatmeal

Preparation time: 10 minutes

Cooking time: 3 hours

Servings: 2

Ingredients:

Cooking spray

2 cups coconut milk

1 cup old fashioned oats

1 pear, cubed

1 apple, cored and cubed 2 tablespoons butter, melted

Directions:

Grease your slow cooker with the cooking spray, add the milk, oats and the other ingredients, toss, put the lid on and cook on High for 3 hours.

Divide the mix into bowls and serve for breakfast.

Nutrition:

Calories 1002,

Fat 74,

Fiber 18,

Carbs 93, Protein 16.2

Egg Casserole

Preparation time: 10 minutes

Cooking time: 6 hours

Servings: 4

Ingredients:

- ¾ cup milk

- ½ teaspoon salt

- 8 large eggs

- ½ teaspoon dry mustard

- ¼ teaspoon black pepper

- 4 cups hash brown potatoes, partially thawed

- ½ cup green bell pepper, chopped

- 4 green onions, chopped

- 12 ounces ham, diced

- ½ cup red bell pepper, chopped 1½ cups cheddar cheese, shredded

Directions:

Whisk together eggs, dry mustard, milk, salt and black pepper in a larg bowl.

Grease the crockpot and put 1/3 of the hash brown potatoes, salt ar black pepper.

ayer with 1/3 of the diced ham, red bell peppers, green bell peppers,
een onions and cheese.

epeat the layers twice, ending with the cheese and top with the egg
ixture.

over and cook on LOW for about 6 hours.

rve this delicious casserole for breakfast.

utrition

lories: 453

t: 26g

rbohydrates: 32.6g

Delish Carrots Oatmeal

Preparation time: 10 minutes

Cooking time: 8 hours

Servings: 2

Ingredients:

- ½ cup old fashioned oats
- 1 cup almond milk
- 2 carrots, peeled and grated
- ½ teaspoon cinnamon powder
- 2 tablespoons brown sugar
- ¼ cup walnuts, chopped
- Cooking spray

Directions:

Grease your slow cooker with cooking spray, add the oats, milk, carro
and the other ingredients, toss, put the lid on and cook on Low for 8 hou

Divide the oatmeal into 2 bowls and serve.

Nutrition:

Calories 590, Fat 40.7,

Fiber 9.1, Carbs 49.9, Protein 12

Cheesy Breakfast Potatoes

Preparation time: 20 minutes

Cooking time: 5 hours

Servings: 6

Ingredients:

1 green bell pepper, diced

1½ cups cheddar cheese, shredded

1 can cream of mushroom soup

4 medium russet potatoes, peeled and diced

1 small yellow onion, diced

4 Andouille sausages, diced

¼ cup sour cream

1/3 cup water

1 teaspoon salt

¼ cup fresh parsley, chopped

1 teaspoon black pepper 1 teaspoon garlic powder

Directions:

Mix together soup, sour cream, water, black pepper, season salt and garlic powder in a one pot crock pot until completely combined.

Top with cheddar cheese and diced vegetables and stir well.

Cover and cook on LOW for about 5 hours.

Dish out and season with more salt and pepper if desired.

Nutrition

Calories: 479

Fat: 29.6g

Carbohydrates: 32g

Apple with Chia Mix

Preparation time: 10 minutes

Cooking time: 8 hours

Servings: 2

Ingredients:

¼ cup chia seeds

2 apples, cored and roughly cubed

1 cup almond milk

2 tablespoons maple syrup

1 teaspoon vanilla extract

½ tablespoon cinnamon powder

Cooking spray

Directions:

Grease your slow cooker with the cooking spray, add the chia seeds, milk and the other ingredients, toss, put the lid on and cook on Low for 8 hours.

Divide the mix into bowls and serve for breakfast.

Nutrition:

Calories 453,

Fat 29.3, Fiber 8, Carbs 51.1, Protein 3.4

Pumpkin pie with sorghum

Preparation time: 10 minutes

Cooking time: 8 hours

Servings: 4

Ingredients:

- Pumpkin pie spice-1 tbsp.

- Maple syrup-2 tbsp. s.

- Vanilla extract-1 tsp.

- Almond milk (unsweetened) - 1 cup

- Sorghum-1 cup

- Pumpkin puree-3/4 cup

Directions:

In a slow cooker combine all the above ingredients and mix well.

Add two cups of water to it and mix again.

Let the mixture cook for 8 hours so that the sorghum gets tender and th liquid gets dissolved.

Serve hot.

Nutrition:

Calories: 221, Total fat: 3g, Cholesterol: 0mg,

Sodium: 52 mg, Carbohydrate: 27g, Dietary fiber: 5g, Protein: 6g

Colorful breakfast dish

Preparation time: 15 minutes

Cooking time: 8 hours

Servings: 12

Ingredients:

1/2 pound bulk crumbled Italian sausage 2 green onions

2 minced cloves garlic

1 chopped red bell pepper

18 eggs

1 cup almond milk

1 tsp. garlic powder 1 tsp. dried oregano

Black pepper

Directions:

Make sure to grease the slow cooker well before starting to use it.

Cook the Italian sausage first, with the green onions and garlic in a separate skillet for about 10-12 minutes. Drain the meat fat.

In the slow cooker, add the sausage, onions and garlic as well as the bell peppers.

In a separate bowl, combine the eggs, coconut milk, and all seasonings.

Cover the slow cooker and cook for about 6-8 hours. Serve warm.

Nutrition:

5 Cal, 11.5 g total fat (3.6 g sat. fat), 172 mg chop. 119 mg sodium,

g carb. 4g fiber, 11.2g protein.

Sugary German Oatmeal

Preparation time: 10 minutes

Cooking time: 8 hours

Servings: 2

Ingredients:

- Cooking spray

- 1 cup steel cut oats

- 3 cups water

- 6 ounces coconut milk

- 2 tablespoons cocoa powder

- 1 tablespoon brown sugar 1 tablespoon coconut, shredded

Directions:

Grease your slow cooker with cooking spray, add oats, water, milk, coc
powder, sugar and shredded coconut, stir, cover and cook on Low for
hours.

Stir oatmeal one more time, divide into 2 bowls and serve for breakfas

Enjoy!

Nutrition:

Calories 200,

Fat 4, Fiber 5, Carbs 17, Protein 5

Cranberry Apple Oats

Preparation time: 10 minutes

Cooking time: 3 hours

Servings: 2

Ingredients:

Cooking spray

2 cups water

1 cup old fashioned oats

¼ cup cranberries, dried

1 apple, chopped

1 tablespoon butter, melted ½ teaspoon cinnamon powder

Directions:

Grease your slow cooker with cooking spray, add water, oats, cranberries, apple, butter and cinnamon, stir well, cover and cook on Low for 3 hours.

Stir oatmeal again, divide into bowls and serve for breakfast.

Enjoy!

Nutrition:

Calories 182,

4, Fiber 6, Carbs 8, Protein 10

Sausage and Potato Mix

Preparation time: 10 minutes

Cooking time: 6 hours

Servings: 2

Ingredients:

- 2 sweet potatoes, peeled and roughly cubed
- 1 green bell pepper, minced
- ½ yellow onion, chopped
- 4 ounces smoked Andouille sausage, sliced
- 1 cup cheddar cheese, shredded
- ¼ cup Greek yogurt
- ¼ teaspoon basil, dried
- 1 cup chicken stock
- Salt and black pepper to the taste
- 1 tablespoon parsley, chopped

Directions:

In your slow cooker, combine the potatoes with the bell pepper, sausa and the other ingredients, toss, put the lid on and cook on Low for 6 hou

Divide between plates and serve for breakfast.

Nutrition:

Calories 623,

Fat 35.7, Fiber 7.6, Carbs 53.1, Protein 24.8

Apple pie oatmeal

Preparation time: 20 minutes

Cooking time: 9 hours

Servings: 4

Ingredients:

Apples (peeled & diced) – 2

Old fashioned oats – 1 cup

Protein powder – ½ cup

Cinnamon – 1 teaspoon

Apple pie spice – ½ teaspoon

Salt – ½ teaspoon

Unsweetened applesauce – ½ cup

Unsweetened almond milk – ½ cup

Low-sugar maple syrup – 2 tablespoon Sweetener of choice – ¼ cup

Directions:-

Combine all the ingredients in a slow cooker.

Cook covered for 6-9 hours on low.

Stir well.

Nutrition:

5 Cal, 4 g

total fat (0 g sat. fat), 35 g carb.

fiber, 13 g protein.

Carrots and Zucchini Oatmeal

Preparation time: 10 minutes

Cooking time: 8 hours

Servings: 2

Ingredients:

- ½ cup steel cut oats
- 1 cup coconut milk
- 1 carrot, grated
- ¼ zucchini, grated
- A pinch of nutmeg, ground
- A pinch of cloves, ground
- ½ teaspoon cinnamon powder
- 2 tablespoons brown sugar
- ¼ cup pecans, chopped
- Cooking spray

Directions:

Grease your slow cooker with cooking spray, add oats, milk, carrc zucchini, nutmeg, cloves, cinnamon and sugar, toss, cover and cook c Low for 8 hours.

Divide into 2 bowls, sprinkle pecans on top and serve.

Enjoy!

Nutrition:

Calories 200, Fat 4, Fiber 8, Carbs 11, Protein 5

Quinoa Spinach Casserole

Preparation time: 10 minutes

Cooking time: 4 hours

Servings: 2

Ingredients:

¼ cup quinoa

1 cup milk

2 eggs

A pinch of salt and black pepper

¼ cup spinach, chopped

¼ cup cherry tomatoes, halved

2 tablespoons cheddar cheese, shredded

2 tablespoons parmesan, shredded

Cooking spray

Directions:

In a bowl, mix eggs **with quinoa**, milk, salt, pepper, tomatoes, spinach and cheddar cheese and whisk well.

Grease your slow cooker with cooking spray, add eggs and quinoa mix, spread parmesan all over, cover and cook on High for 4 hours.

Divide between plates and serve.

Enjoy!

Nutrition:

Calories 251, Fat 5, Fiber 7, Carbs 19, Protein 11

Coconut Quinoa Mix

Preparation time: 10 minutes

Cooking time: 8 hours

Servings: 2

Ingredients:

- ½ cup quinoa

- 1 cup water

- ½ cup coconut milk

- 1 tablespoon maple syrup

- A pinch of salt 1 tablespoon berries

Directions:

In your slow cooker, mix quinoa with water, coconut milk, maple syr
and salt, stir well, cover and cook on Low for 8 hours.

Divide into 2 bowls, sprinkle berries on top and serve for breakfast.

Enjoy!

Nutrition:

Calories 261,

Fat 5, Fiber 7, Carbs 12, Protein 5

Milky Apple Oatmeal

Preparation time: 10 minutes

Cooking time: 8 hours

Servings: 2

Ingredients:

½ cup steel cut oats

1 apple, chopped 1 cup apple juice

1 cup milk

2 tablespoons maple syrup

1 teaspoon vanilla extract

½ tablespoon cinnamon powder

A pinch of nutmeg, ground

Cooking spray

Directions:

Grease your slow cooker with the cooking spray, add oats, apple, apple juice, milk, maple syrup, vanilla extract, cinnamon and nutmeg, stir, cover and cook on Low for 8 hours.

Stir oatmeal one more time, divide into bowls and serve.

Enjoy!

Nutrition:

Calories 221,

Fat 4, Fiber 6, Carbs 8, Protein 10

Veggie Hash Brown Mix

Preparation time: 10 minutes

Cooking time: 6 hours and 5 minutes

Servings: 2

Ingredients:

- 1 tablespoon olive oil
- ½ cup white mushrooms, chopped
- ½ yellow onion, chopped
- ¼ teaspoon garlic powder ¼ teaspoon onion powder
- ¼ cup sour cream
- 10 ounces hash browns
- ¼ cup cheddar cheese, shredded
- Salt and black pepper to the taste ½ tablespoon parsley, chopped

Directions:

Heat up a pan with the oil over medium heat, add the onion and mushroom stir and cook for 5 minutes.

Transfer this to the slow cooker, add hash browns and the other ingredien toss, put the lid on and cook on Low for 6 hours.

Divide between plates and for breakfast.

Nutrition:

Calories 571,

Fat 35.6, Fiber 5.4, Carbs 54.9, Protein 9.7

Banana oatmeal

Preparation time: 5 minutes

Cooking time: 8 hours

Servings: 4

Ingredients:

Steel cut oats – 1 cup

Mashed ripe banana – 1

Chopped walnuts – ¼ cup

Skim milk – 2 cups

Water – 2 cups

Flax seed meal – 2 tablespoon

Cinnamon – 2 teaspoon

Vanilla – 1 teaspoon

Nutmeg – ½ teaspoon

Salt – ½ teaspoon

Banana slices – for garnish

Chopped walnuts – for garnish

Directions:-

Combine all the ingredients in a slow cooker except the banana slices and walnuts.

Cook covered for 8 hours on low.

Stir well.

Serve topped with walnuts and banana slices.

Nutrition:

290 Cal,

8 g total fat (7 g sat. fat),

2 mg cholesterol,

366 mg sodium, 42 g carb.

6.6g fiber,

11 g protein.

Cheesy Tater Tot Casserole

Preparation time: 10 minutes

Cooking time: 4 hours

Servings: 2

Ingredients:

Cooking spray

10 ounces tater tots, frozen

2 eggs, whisked

½ pound turkey sausage, ground

1 tablespoon heavy cream

¼ teaspoon thyme, dried

¼ teaspoon garlic powder

A pinch of salt and black pepper ½ cup Colby jack cheese, shredded

Directions:

Grease your slow cooker with cooking spray, spread tater tots on the bottom, add sausage, thyme, garlic powder, salt, pepper and whisked eggs.

Add cheese, cover pot and cook on Low for 4 hours.

Divide between plates and serve for breakfast.

Enjoy!

Nutrition:

Calories 231,

5, Fiber 9, Carbs 15, Protein 11

Cheddar & Bacon Casserole

Preparation time: 10 minutes

Cooking time: 3 hours

Servings: 2

Ingredients:

- 5 ounces hash browns, shredded
- 2 bacon slices, cooked and chopped
- 2 ounces cheddar cheese, shredded
- 3 eggs, whisked
- 1 green onion, chopped
- ¼ cup milk
- Cooking spray
- A pinch of salt and black pepper

Directions:

Grease your slow cooker with cooking spray and add hash browns, bac
and cheese.

In a bowl, mix eggs with green onion, milk, salt and pepper, whisk w
and add to slow cooker.

Cover, cook on High for 3 hours, divide between plates and serve.

Enjoy!

Nutrition:

Calories 281, Fat 4, Fiber 6, Carbs 12, Protein 11

Breakfast turkey meatloaf

Preparation time: 10 minutes

Cooking time: 4 hours

Servings: 6

Ingredients:

2 pounds ground turkey

1 chopped small red onion

2 minced cloves garlic

1 tsp. garlic powder 1 tsp. dried oregano

1 tsp. dried basil

¼ cup coconut flour

Salt and pepper

2 eggs

Coconut oil

Directions:

Heat some coconut oil in a skillet, cook the garlic and onion for 5 minutes. Set aside.

Add the ground turkey in a bowl with the garlic, onions, and all spices. Use your hands to mix thoroughly.

Shape the meat as a loaf and place it in the bottom of the slow cooker.

Cook for about 3.5 hours.

Serve with your favorite homemade ketchup.

Nutrition:

195 Cal,

7.5 g total fat (1.6 g sat. fat),

102 mg cholesterol

119 mg sodium,

5.5 g carb.

5g fiber,

9.2g protein.

Broccoli Casserole

Preparation time: 10 minutes

Cooking time: 6 hours

Servings: 2

Ingredients:

2 eggs, whisked

1 cup broccoli florets

2 cups hash browns

½ teaspoon coriander, ground

½ teaspoon rosemary, dried

½ teaspoon turmeric powder

½ teaspoon mustard powder

A pinch of salt and black pepper

1 small red onion, chopped ½ red bell pepper, chopped

1 ounce cheddar cheese, shredded

Cooking spray

Directions:

Grease your slow cooker with the cooking spray, and spread hash browns, broccoli, bell pepper and the onion on the bottom of the pan.

In a bowl, mix the eggs with the coriander and the other ingredients, whisk and pour over the broccoli mix in the pot.

Put the lid on, cook on Low for 6 hours, divide between plates and serve for breakfast.

Nutrition:

Calories 261,

Fat 7,

Fiber 8,

Carbs 20,

Protein 11

Pumpkin Oatmeal

Preparation time: 10 minutes

Cooking time: 7 hours

Servings: 2

Ingredients:

Cooking spray

½ cup steel cut oats

1 cup water

1 cup almond milk

1 and ½ tablespoon maple syrup

½ teaspoon vanilla extract

½ teaspoon pumpkin pie spice

½ cup pumpkin, chopped ¼ teaspoon cinnamon powder

Directions:

Grease your slow cooker with cooking spray, add steel cut oats, water, almond milk, maple syrup, vanilla, pumpkin spice, pumpkin and cinnamon, stir, cover and cook on Low for 7 hours.

Stir one more time, divide into bowls and serve.

Enjoy!

Nutrition:

Calories 242,

Fat 3,

Fiber 8, carbs 20, protein 7

Smooth apple butter

Preparation time: 10 minutes

Cooking time: 7 hours

Servings: 4

Ingredients:

- 16-20 dates - cut into halves
- 4 diced apples, peeled and cored
- 1 cup apple cider
- ½ cup molasses
- 2 Tbsp. ground cinnamon
- ½ Tsp. nutmeg

Directions:

Simply place all ingredients in your slow cooker and mix well.

Cook for about 7 hours. The apples should be very tender, so you c
easily blend them in your food processor.

Put actually everything from the slow cooker in the food processor a
activate until the texture is every smooth.

Spread on whatever your heart desires!

Nutrition:

79 Cal, 1.9 g total fat (0.2 g sat. fat), 0 mg chop. 27 mg sodium,

12.5 g carb. 4g fiber, 7.2g protein.

Flavorful Coconut Quinoa

Preparation time: 10 minutes

Cooking time: 8 hours

Servings: 2

Ingredients

- ½ cup quinoa
- 2 cups coconut milk
- 1 tablespoon maple syrup
- 1 teaspoon vanilla extract
- 2 tablespoons raisins
- ¼ cup blackberries

Directions:

In your slow cooker, mix the quinoa with the milk, maple syrup and the other ingredients, toss, put the lid on and cook on Low for 8 hours.

Divide into 2 bowls and serve for breakfast.

Nutrition:

Calories 775,

Fat 60,

Fiber 9.7,

Carbs 56.5, Protein 12

Mexican casserole

Preparation time: 15 minutes

Cooking time: 6 hours

Servings: 4

Ingredients:

- Taco seasoning – 1/2 packets Turkey bacon-1/2 lb. . . .

- Salsa

- Jalapeno chilies

- Mushrooms-8 oz.

- Sweet potato (cubed) - 1

- Red bell pepper-1

- Eggs (whisked) - 8

- Yellow onion (chopped) - 1

- Guacamole

Directions:

In a skillet, fry the turkey bacon and crumble it when cooled.

Fry the onions till they turn soft.

Except for taco seasoning, mix all the ingredients and transfer it to a slow cooker.

Sprinkle the taco seasoning.

Cook for 6 to 8 hours on low setting.

Serve with guacamole, jalapeno chilies and salsa.

Nutrition:

Calories: 430,

Total fat: 26g,

Cholesterol: 480mg,

Sodium: 1570mg,

Carbohydrate: 18g,

Dietary fiber: 4g,

Protein: 33g

Quinoa and Veggies Casserole

Preparation time: 10 minutes

Cooking time: 6 hours

Servings: 2

Ingredients:

- ¼ cup quinoa

- 1 cup almond milk

- 2 eggs, whisked

- 1 tablespoon parsley, chopped

- 1 tablespoon chives, chopped

- A pinch of salt and black pepper

- ¼ cup baby spinach

- ¼ cup cherry tomatoes, halved

- 2 tablespoons parmesan, shredded

- Cooking spray

Directions:

Grease your slow cooker with the cooking spray, add the quinoa mixed with the milk, eggs and the other ingredients except the parmesan, to and spread into the pot.

Sprinkle the parmesan on top, put the lid on and cook on Low for 6 hour

Divide between plates and serve.

Nutrition:

Calories 251, Fat 5, Fiber 7, Carbs 19, Protein 11

Cabbage in the slow cooker

Preparation time: 10 minutes

Cooking time: 6 hours

Servings: 8

Ingredients:

1 head chopped green cabbage

1 chopped leek

3 crushed cloves garlic

¼ cup grass fed butter

Salt and pepper

1 Tbsp. celery seeds

Directions:

First in the slow cooker, melt the butter and then add the leek and garlic and the shredded cabbage.

Stir and then add all spices.

Cover and cook for 6 hours.

When you uncover, you will need to adjust seasonings, probably add salt and pepper for sure.

You can also sprinkle some chopped pecans that would be delicious.

Nutrition:

Cal, 3.5 g total fat (0.6 g sat. fat), 10 mg chop. 69 mg sodium,

g carb. 4.3g fiber, 7.2g protein.

Pumpkin and Quinoa Mix

Preparation time: 10 minutes

Cooking time: 8 hours

Servings: 2

Ingredients:

- Cooking spray
- ½ cup quinoa
- 1 cup almond milk
- 1 tablespoon honey
- ¼ cup pumpkin puree
- ½ teaspoon vanilla extract ¼ teaspoon cinnamon powder

Directions:

Grease your slow cooker with the cooking spray, add the quinoa, mi
honey and the other ingredients, stir, put the lid on and cook on Low
7 hours.

Divide the mix into bowls and serve for breakfast.

Nutrition:

Calories 242,

Fat 3,

Fiber 8, Carbs 20, Protein 7

Cinnamon French toast

Preparation time: 10 minutes

Cooking time: 4 hours

Servings: 2

Ingredients:

½ French baguette, sliced

2 ounces cream cheese

1 tablespoon brown sugar

1 egg, whisked

3 tablespoons almond milk

2 tablespoons honey

½ teaspoon cinnamon powder

1 tablespoon butter, melted Cooking spray

Directions:

Spread the cream cheese on all bread slices, grease your slow cooker with the cooking spray and arrange the slices in the pot.

In a bowl, mix the egg with the cinnamon, almond milk and the remaining ingredients, whisk and pour over the bread slices.

Put the lid on, cook on High for 4 hours, divide the mix between plates and serve for breakfast.

Nutrition:

Calories 316,

23.5, Fiber 0.5, Carbs 23.9, Protein 5.6

Veggies and sausage casserole

Preparation time: 15 minutes

Cooking time: 4 hours

Servings: 6

Ingredients:

- Garlic clot ves-2 tsp.

- Sweet potatoes-23

- Coconut oil – 2 tbsps.

- Eggs-8

- Leeks-1

- Beef sausage-1 ½ cup Kale (chopped) - 1 cup

Directions:

Sauté garlic, leeks and kale in coconut oil in a medium skillet.

In a large bowl combine the remaining ingredients and let it cook for 4 6 hours.

Once cooked, serve.

Nutrition:

Calories: 448,

Total fat: 35g,

Cholesterol: 350mg,

Carbohydrate: 18g,

Dietary fiber: 1g, Sodium: 649 mg, Protein: 25g

Hash Brown with Bacon

Preparation time: 10 minutes

Cooking time: 3 hours

Servings: 2

Ingredients:

5 ounces hash browns, shredded

2 bacon slices, cooked and chopped

¼ cup mozzarella cheese, shredded

2 eggs, whisked

¼ cup sour cream

1 tablespoon cilantro, chopped

1 tablespoon olive oil

A pinch of salt and black pepper

Directions:

Grease your slow cooker with the oil, add the hash browns mixed with the eggs, sour cream and the other ingredients, toss, put the lid on and cook on High for 4 hours.

Divide the casserole into bowls and serve.

Nutrition:

Calories 383, Fat 26.9,

Fiber 2.3, Carbs 26.6, Protein 9.6

Cinnamon Oatmeal

Preparation time: 10 minutes

Cooking time: 6 hours

Servings: 2

Ingredients:

- 1 cup old fashioned oats

- 1 cup blackberries

- 3 cups almond milk

- ½ cup Greek yogurt

- ½ teaspoon cinnamon powder ½ teaspoon vanilla extract

Directions:

In your slow cooker, mix the oats with the milk, berries and the other ingredients, toss, put the lid on and cook on Low for 6 hours.

Divide into bowls and serve for breakfast.

Nutrition:

Calories 932,

Fat 43,

Fiber 16.7,

Carbs 82.2,

Protein 24.3

CONCLUSION

Thank you for making it through to the end of our book. Let's hope it was informative and able to provide you with all of the tools you need to achieve your goals in weight loss and a healthier lifestyle. Now that you are familiar with the Keto diet on many levels, you should feel confident in your ability to start your own Keto journey. This diet plan isn't going to hinder you or limit you, so do your best to keep this in mind as you begin changing your lifestyle and adjusting your eating habits. Packed with plenty of proteins and good fats your body is going to go through a transformation as it works to see these things as energy. Before you know it, your body will have an automatically accessible reserve that you can utilize. Whether you need a boost of energy first thing in the morning or a second wind to keep you going throughout the day, this will already be inside of you.

CPSIA information can be obtained
at www.ICGtesting.com
Printed in the USA
BVHW062042040521
606420BV00010B/2269

9 781802 570748